DIABETIC COOKBOOK FOR BEGINNERS 2021

JESSICA TAYLOR

DISCLAIMER

The information contained in the Book is for informational purposes only, and in no case may it constitute the formulation of a diagnosis or the prescription of treatment.
The information contained in the Book is not intended and should not in any way replace the direct doctor-patient relationship or the specialist visit.
It is recommended to always seek the advice of your doctor and/ or specialists regarding any indication reported.

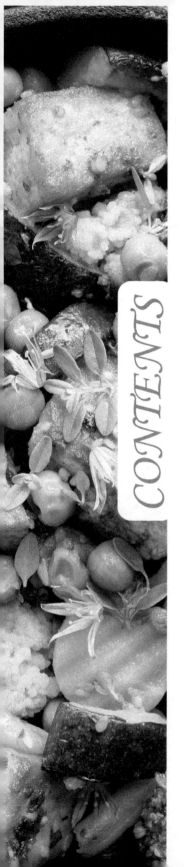

CONTENTS

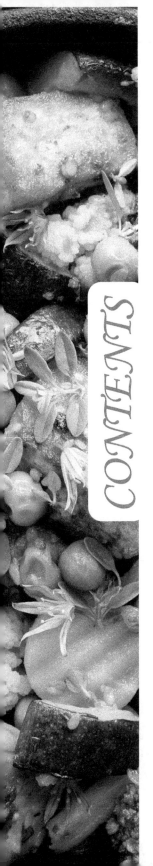

CONTENTS

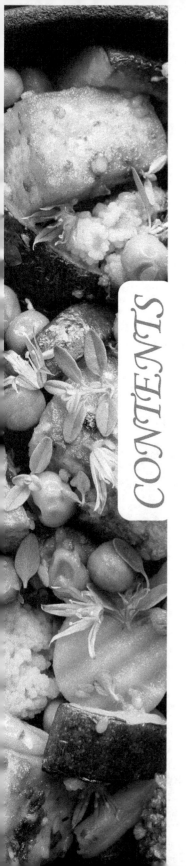

CONTENTS

INTRODUCTION

For sure, discovering that you have diabetes is not good news, you may feel as if all your certainties are collapsing, especially about health, even more so if diabetes creeps into you out of nowhere. You may no longer feel in control of your life and use this feeling as an excuse to "let go".

Know that this state of mind is YOUR choice, some people live with diabetes without problems and live great! I don't see why you should be outdone. You will have to start taking your life in hand and dedicate yourself to yourself!

YOU CAN MANAGE DIABETES! Start repeating this phrase until you are convinced and from there you can finally start a new life, it works!

Once you know the benefits of certain methods, such as avoiding pitfalls and adapting to changes that improve your health, there is no reason in the world why you cannot live on your terms and be incredibly happy and healthy at all. same time!

By keeping your blood sugar as close to your goal as possible, you will be able to prevent or delay diabetes-related complications, which is the main reason we all fear when diagnosed.

By simply checking your blood sugar levels and adjusting where possible (the key to this is knowing what can be changed!), You'll soon see that diabetes doesn't have to be the monster you originally thought it was.

Whether you have type 1 diabetes (insulin deficiency) or type 2 diabetes (insulin resistance), diabetes is the result of excess blood sugar. If left unchecked, it will overwhelm your kidneys and will spill into your urine.

The high blood sugar level can also damage the nerves, creating the condition of neuropathy. This damage shows signs of numbness, tingling, and pain. Poor circulation can also develop, leaving a lack of sensation in the extremities, which can eventually lead to poorly healing wounds and end up as amputations.

Diabetes has tripled in the past 30 years, with over 20 million

Americans being diagnosed with type 1 (5% to 10% of cases) or type 2 (90% to 95% of cases) diabetes) [1].

I don't mean to scare you with these facts, but knowing them will help you deviate from temptations along the way. If you don't heed the warnings and tweak the harmful damage, you may simply have justified the fear you originally felt.

The main reason your cells cannot assimilate the sugars they need to create energy and regenerate cells and growth is that they have developed a sticky substance that resists insulin (type 2 diabetes).

The good news is that type 1 diabetes is regulated by insulin, which rebuilds insulin for use in cells. Type 2 diabetes can also be regulated with medication, but the best and healthiest way is with an active lifestyle and a nutritious diet. You are in control of both of these things, so let's not get lost in small talk and get started right away!

BENEFITS OF PHYSICAL EXERCISE!

You should consider exercise, especially if aerobic, is an integral part of your diabetes treatment plan and should include at least 30 minutes of walking per day (or another form of exercise) for a total of three hours of exercise per week.

Regular physical activity, in fact, not only helps to fight stress but also has important beneficial effects on metabolism: it improves insulin sensitivity, reduces triglyceride and bad cholesterol levels (Ldl) to the advantage of the good one (HDL), helps control blood pressure and prevents cardiovascular disease.

On the other hand, sports with a high risk of trauma, especially at the head level, should be avoided in some patients.

Veggie and Tofu Stir-Fry

Preparation Time: 10 minutes | Cooking Time: 10 minutes | Servings: 4

- 3 tablespoons extra-virgin olive oil

- 12 ounces (340 g) firm tofu, cut into ½-inch pieces

- 4 cups broccoli, broken into florets

- 4 scallions, sliced

- 1 teaspoon peeled and grated fresh ginger

- 4 garlic cloves, minced

- 2 tablespoons soy sauce (use gluten-free soy sauce if necessary)

- ¼ cup vegetable broth

- 1 cup cooked brown rice

Heat the olive oil in a large skillet over medium-high heat until simmering.

Add the tofu, broccoli, and scallions and stir fry for 6 minutes, or until the vegetables start to become tender.

Add the ginger and garlic and cook for about 30 seconds, stirring constantly.

Fold in the soy sauce, vegetable broth, and brown rice. Stir to combine and cook for an additional 1 to 2 minutes until the rice is heated through.

Let it cool for 5 minutes before serving.

Nutritional Info:

Calories: 238 | fat: 13.2g

Protein: 11.1g | carbs: 21.2g

Fiber: 4.2g | saturated fat: 2g

Sodium:360 mg

Vegetable Stuffed Portobello Mushrooms

Preparation Time: 5 minutes | Cooking Time: 20 minutes | Servings: 4

- 8 large portobello mushrooms

- 3 teaspoons extra-virgin olive oil, divided

- 4 cups fresh spinach

- 1 medium red bell pepper, diced

- ¼ cup feta cheese, crumbled

Preheat the oven to 450°F (235°C).

On your cutting board, remove the mushroom stems. Scoop out the gills with a spoon and discard. Grease the mushrooms with 2 tablespoons olive oil.

Arrange the mushrooms, cap-side down, on a baking sheet. Roast in the preheated oven for 20 minutes until browned on top.

Meanwhile, in a skillet, heat the remaining olive oil over medium heat until shimmering.

Add the spinach and red bell pepper to the skillet and sauté for 8 minutes until the vegetables are tender, stirring occasionally. Remove from the heat to a bowl.

Remove the mushrooms from the oven to a plate. Using a spoon to stuff the mushrooms with the vegetables and sprinkle with the feta cheese. Serve warm.

Nutritional Info:

Calories: 118

Fat: 6.3g

Protein: 7.2g

Carbs: 12.2g

Fiber: 4.1g

Sugar: 6.1g

Sodium: 128mg

Vegetable Baked Eggs

Preparation Time: 5 minutes | Cooking Time: 25 minutes | Servings: 4

- 2 tablespoons extra-virgin olive oil

- 1 red onion, chopped

- 1 sweet potato, cut into ½-inch pieces

- 1 green bell pepper, seeded and chopped

- ½ teaspoon sea salt

- 1 teaspoon chili powder

- 4 large eggs

- ½ cup shredded pepper Jack cheese

- 1 avocado, cut into cubes

Preheat the oven to 350°F (180°C).

Heat the olive oil in a large skillet over medium-high heat until shimmering.

Add the onion, sweet potato, bell pepper, salt, and chili powder. Cook for about 10 minutes, stirring constantly, or until the vegetables are lightly browned.

Remove from the heat. With the back of a spoon, make 4 wells in the vegetables, then crack an egg into each well. Scatter the shredded cheese over the vegetables.

Bake in the preheated oven for about 10 minutes until the cheese is melted and eggs are set.

Remove from the heat and sprinkle the avocado on top before serving.

Nutritional Info:

Calories: 286

Fat: 21.3g

Protein: 12.3g

Carbs: 16.2g

Fiber: 5.2g

Saturated fat g

Sodium: 266mg

Sautéed Collard Greens and Cabbage

Preparation Time: 10 minutes | Cooking Time: 10 minutes | Servings: 8

- 2 tablespoons extra-virgin olive oil
- 1 collard greens bunch, stemmed and thinly sliced
- ½ small green cabbage, thinly sliced
- 6 garlic cloves, minced
- 1 tablespoon low-sodium soy sauce

Heat the olive oil in a large skillet over medium-high heat.

Sauté the collard greens in the oil for about 2 minutes, or until the greens start to wilt.

Toss in the cabbage and mix well. Reduce the heat to medium-low, cover, and cook for 5 to 7 minutes, stirring occasionally, or until the greens are softened.

Fold in the garlic and soy sauce and stir to combine. Cook for about 30 seconds more until fragrant.

Remove from the heat to a plate and serve.

Nutritional Info:

calories: 73 | fat: 4.1g | protein: 3.2g | carbs: 5.9g | fiber: 2.9g | sugar: 0g | sodium: 128mg

Simple Sautéed Greens

Preparation Time: 10 minutes | Cooking Time: 10 minutes | Servings: 4

- 2 tablespoons extra-virgin olive oil
- 1 pound (454 g) Swiss chard, coarse stems removed and leaves chopped
- 1 pound (454 g) kale, coarse stems removed and leaves chopped
- ½ teaspoon ground cardamom
- 1 tablespoon freshly squeezed lemon juice
- Sea salt and freshly ground black pepper, to taste

Heat the olive oil in a large skillet over medium-high heat.

Add the Swiss chard, kale, cardamon, and lemon juice to the skillet, and stir to combine. Cook for about 10 minutes, stirring continuously, or until the greens are wilted.

Sprinkle with the salt and pepper and stir well.

Serve the greens on a plate while warm.

Nutritional Info:

calories: 139 | fat: 6.8g | protein: 5.9g | carbs: 15.8g | fiber: 3.9g | sugar: 1.0g | sodium: 350mg

Sesame Bok Choy with Almonds

Preparation Time: 15 minutes | Cooking Time: 7 minutes | Servings: 4

- 2 teaspoons sesame oil

- 2 pounds (907 g) bok choy, cleaned and quartered

- 2 teaspoons low-sodium soy sauce

- Pinch red pepper flakes

- ½ cup toasted sliced almonds

Heat the sesame oil in a large skillet over medium heat until hot.

Sauté the bok choy in the hot oil for about 5 minutes, stirring occasionally, or until tender but still crisp.

Add the soy sauce and red pepper flakes and stir to combine. Continue sautéing for 2 minutes.

Transfer to a plate and serve topped with sliced almonds.

Nutritional Info:

calories: 118 | fat: 7.8g | protein: 6.2g | carbs: 7.9g | fiber: 4.1g | sugar: 3.0g | sodium: 293mg

Garlicky Mushrooms

Preparation Time: 10 minutes | Cooking Time: 12 minutes | Servings: 4

- 1 tablespoon butter

- 2 teaspoons extra-virgin olive oil

- 2 pounds (907 g) button mushrooms, halved

- 2 teaspoons minced fresh garlic

- 1 teaspoon chopped fresh thyme

- Sea salt and freshly ground black pepper, to taste

Heat the butter and olive oil in a large skillet over medium-high heat.

Add the mushrooms and sauté for 10 minutes, stirring occasionally, or until the mushrooms are lightly browned and cooked though.

Stir in the garlic and thyme and cook for an additional 2 minutes.

Season with salt and pepper and serve on a plate.

Nutritional Info:

calories: 96 | fat: 6.1g | protein: 6.9g | carbs: 8.2g | fiber: 1.7g | sugar: 3.9g | sodium: 91mg

Italian Eggplant Rollups

Preparation Time: 10 minutes | Cooking Time: 50 minutes | Servings: 8

- 16 fresh spinach leaves

- 4 sun-dried tomatoes, rinsed, drained and diced fine

- 2 medium eggplants

- 1 green onion, diced fine

- 4 tablespoons fat-free cream cheese, soft

- 2 tablespoons fat-free sour cream

- 2 tablespoons lemon juice

- 1 teaspoon olive oil

- 1 clove garlic, diced fine

- ¼ teaspoon oregano

- ⅛ teaspoon black pepper

- Nonstick cooking spray

- Spaghetti Sauce:

- ½ onion, diced

- ½ carrot, grated

- ½ stalk celery, diced

- ½ zucchini, grated

- ½ (28-ounce / 794-g) Italian-style tomatoes, in puree

- ½ (14½-ounce / 411-g) diced tomatoes, with juice

- ¼ cup water

- 1 clove garlic, diced fine

- ¼ tablespoon oregano

- ½ teaspoon olive oil

- ½ teaspoon basil

- ½ teaspoon thyme

- ½ teaspoon salt

- ¼ teaspoon red pepper flakes

Heat oven to 450°F (235°C). Spray 2 large cookie sheets with cooking spray.

Trim the ends of the eggplant. Slice them lengthwise in ¼-inch slices. Discard the ones that are mostly skin, there should be about 16 slices. Arrange them in a single layer on prepared pans.

In a small bowl, whisk together the lemon juice and oil and brush over both sides of the eggplant. Bake 20 to 25 minutes or until the eggplant starts to turn a golden brown color. Transfer to a plate to cool.

Meanwhile, make the spaghetti sauce: Heat oil in a large saucepan over medium heat. Add vegetables and garlic. Cook, stirring frequently, until vegetables get soft, about 5 minutes.

Add remaining Ingredients, use the back of a spoon to break up tomatoes. Bring to a simmer and cook, partially covered, over medium-low heat for 30 minutes, stirring frequently.

In a mixing bowl, combine remaining , except spinach, until thoroughly combined.

To assemble, spread 1 teaspoon cream cheese mixture evenly over sliced eggplant, leaving ½-inch border around the edges .Top with a spinach leaf and roll up, starting at small end. Lay rolls, seam side down, on serving plate. Serve with warm spaghetti sauce.

Nutritional Info:

calories: 80 | fat: 3.0g | protein: 3.2g | carbs: 12.1g | fiber: 6.0g | sugar: 6.0g | sodium: 263mg

Roasted Tomato Brussels Sprouts

Preparation Time: 15 minutes | Cooking Time: 20 minutes | Servings: 4

- 1 pound (454 g) Brussels sprouts, trimmed and halved

- 1 tablespoon extra-virgin olive oil

- Sea salt and freshly ground black pepper, to taste

- ½ cup sun-dried tomatoes, chopped

- 2 tablespoons freshly squeezed lemon juice

- 1 teaspoon lemon zest

Preheat the oven to 400°F (205°C). Line a large baking sheet with aluminum foil.

Toss the Brussels sprouts in the olive oil in a large bowl until well coated. Sprinkle with salt and pepper.

Spread out the seasoned Brussels sprouts on the prepared baking sheet in a single layer.

Roast in the preheated oven for 20 minutes, shaking the pan halfway through, or until the Brussels sprouts are crispy and browned on the outside.

Remove from the oven to a serving bowl. Add the tomatoes, lemon juice, and lemon zest, and stir to incorporate. Serve immediately.

Nutritional Info:

Calories: 111

Fat: 5.8g

Protein: 5.0g

Carbs: 13.7g

Fiber: 4.9g

Sugar: 2.7g

Sodium: 103mg

Lime Asparagus with Cashews

Preparation Time: 10 minutes | Cooking Time: 15 to 20 minutes | Servings: 4

- 2 pounds (907 g) asparagus, woody ends trimmed

- 1 tablespoon extra-virgin olive oil

- Sea salt and freshly ground black pepper, to taste

- ½ cup chopped cashews

- Zest and juice of 1 lime

Preheat the oven to 400°F (205°C). Line a baking sheet with aluminum foil.

Toss the asparagus with the olive oil in a medium bowl. Sprinkle the salt and pepper to season.

Arrange the asparagus on the baking sheet and bake for 15 to 20 minutes, or until lightly browned and tender.

Remove the asparagus from the oven to a serving bowl. Add the cashews, lime zest and juice, and toss to coat well. Serve immediately.

Nutritional Info:

calories: 173 | fat: 11.8g | protein: 8.0g | carbs: 43.7g | fiber: 4.9g | sugar: 5.0g | sodium: 65mg

Mini Spinach Quiches

Preparation Time: 10 minutes | Cooking Time: 15 minutes | Servings: 6

- 2 tablespoons olive oil, divided

- 1 onion, finely chopped

- 2 garlic cloves, minced

- 2 cups baby spinach

- 8 large eggs

- ¼ cup whole milk

- ½ teaspoon sea salt

- ¼ teaspoon freshly ground black pepper

- 1 cup Swiss cheese, shredded

Special Equipment:

A 6-cup muffin tin

Preheat the oven to 375°F (190°C). Grease a 6-cup muffin tin with 1 tablespoon olive oil.

Heat the olive oil in a nonstick skillet over medium-high heat.

Add the onion and garlic to the skillet and sauté for 4 minutes until translucent.

Add the spinach to the skillet and sauté for 1 minute until tender. Transfer them to a plate and set aside.

Whisk together the eggs, milk, salt, and black pepper in a bowl.

Dunk the cooked vegetables in the bowl of egg mixture, then scatter with the cheese.

Divide the mixture among the muffin cups. Bake in the preheated oven for 15 minutes until puffed and the edges are golden brown.

Transfer the quiches to six small plates and serve warm.

Nutritional Info:

calories: 220 | fat: 17.2g | protein: 14.3g | carbs: 4.2g | fiber: 0.8g | saturated fat: 6g | sodium: 235mg

Citrus Sautéed Spinach

Servings: 4

Cooking Time: 5 Minutes

Ingredients:

- 2 tablespoons extra-virgin olive oil

- 4 cups fresh baby spinach

- 1 teaspoon orange zest

- ¼ cup freshly squeezed orange juice

- ½ teaspoon sea salt

- ⅛ teaspoon freshly ground black pepper

Directions:

In a large skillet over medium-high heat, heat the olive oil until it shimmers.

Add the spinach and orange zest. Cook for about 3 minutes, stirring occasionally, until the spinach wilts.

Stir in the orange juice, sea salt, and pepper. Cook for 2 minutes more, stirring occasionally. Serve hot.

Nutrition Info:

Calories: 74; Protein: 7g; Total Carbohydrates: 3g; Sugars: 1g; Fiber: 1g; Total Fat: 7g; Saturated Fat: 1g;Cholesterol: 0mg;Sodium: 258mg

Popcorn Style Cauliflower

Preparation Time: 5 minutes | Cooking Time: 20 minutes | Servings: 4

- 1 head cauliflower, separated into bite-sized florets

- ¼ teaspoon garlic powder

- ¼ teaspoon salt

- ⅛ teaspoon black pepper

- Butter-flavored cooking spray

Heat oven to 400°F (205°C).

Place cauliflower in a large bowl and spray with cooking spray, making sure to coat all sides. Sprinkle with seasonings and toss to coat.

Place in a single layer on a cookie sheet. Bake for 20 to 25 minutes or until cauliflower starts to brown. Serve warm.

Nutritional Info:

calories: 55 | fat: 0g | protein: 4.2g | carbs: 11.1g | fiber: 5.0g | sugar: 5.0g | sodium: 165mg

Pesto Stuffed Mushrooms

Preparation Time: 5 minutes | Cooking Time: 20 minutes | Servings: 4

- 12 cremini mushrooms, stems removed
- 4 ounces (113 g) low fat cream cheese, soft
- ½ cup Mozzarella cheese, grated
- ⅓ cup reduced fat Parmesan cheese
- 6 tablespoons basil pesto
- Nonstick cooking spray

Heat oven to 375°F (190°C). Line a square baking dish with foil and spray with cooking spray. Arrange the mushrooms in the baking pan. Set aside.

In a medium bowl, beat cream cheese, pesto and Parmesan until smooth and creamy. Spoon mixture into mushroom caps. Top with a heaping teaspoon of Mozzarella.

Bake 20 to 23 minutes or until cheese is melted and golden brown. Let cook 5 to 10 minutes before serving.

Nutritional Info:

calories: 77 | fat: 3.0g | protein: 8.2g | carbs: 4.1g | fiber: 0g | sugar: 1.0g | sodium: 541mg

Easy Brussels Sprouts Hash

Servings: 4

Cooking Time: 10 Minutes

Ingredients:

- 3 tablespoons extra-virgin olive oil

- 1 onion, finely chopped

- 1 pound Brussels sprouts, bottoms trimmed off, shredded (see tip)

- ½ teaspoon caraway seeds

- ½ teaspoon sea salt

- ⅛ teaspoon freshly ground black pepper

- ¼ cup red wine vinegar

- 1 tablespoon Dijon mustard

- 1 tablespoon honey

- 3 garlic cloves, minced

Directions:

In a large skillet over medium-high heat, heat the olive oil until it shimmers.

Add the onion, Brussels sprouts, caraway seeds, sea salt, and pepper. Cook for 7 to 10 minutes, stirring occasionally, until the Brussels sprouts begin to brown.

While the Brussels sprouts cook, whisk the vinegar, mustard, and honey in a small bowl and set aside.

Add the garlic to the skillet and cook for 30 seconds, stirring constantly.

Add the vinegar mixture to the skillet. Cook for about 5 minutes, stirring, until the liquid reduces by half.

Nutrition Info:

Calories: 176; Protein: 11g

Total Carbohydrates: 19g; Sugars: 8g

Fiber: 5g; Total Fat: 11g

Saturated Fat: 1g; Cholesterol: 0mg

Sodium: 309mg

Simple Parmesan Acorn Squash

Preparation Time: 10 minutes | Cooking Time: 20 minutes | Servings: 4

- 1 acorn squash (about 1 pound / 454 g)

- 1 tablespoon extra-virgin olive oil

- 1 teaspoon dried sage leaves, crumbled

- ¼ teaspoon freshly grated nutmeg

- ⅛ teaspoon kosher salt

- ⅛ teaspoon freshly ground black pepper

- 2 tablespoons freshly grated Parmesan cheese

Cut the acorn squash in half lengthwise and remove the seeds. Cut each half in half for a total of 4 wedges. Snap off the stem if it's easy to do.

In a small bowl, combine the olive oil, sage, nutmeg, salt, and pepper. Brush the cut sides of the squash with the olive oil mixture.

Pour 1 cup of water into the electric pressure cooker and insert a wire rack or trivet.

Place the squash on the trivet in a single layer, skin-side down.

Close and lock the lid of the pressure cooker. Set the valve to sealing.

Cook on high pressure for 20 minutes.

When the cooking is complete, hit Cancel and quick release the pressure.

Once the pin drops, unlock and remove the lid.

Carefully remove the squash from the pot, sprinkle with the Parmesan, and serve.

Nutritional Info:

calories: 86 | fat: 4.1g | protein: 2.1g | carbs: 11.9g | fiber: 2.1g | sugar: 0g | sodium: 283mg

Tarragon Spring Peas

Preparation Time: 10 minutes | Cooking Time: 12 minutes | Servings: 6 (½ cup each)

- 1 tablespoon unsalted butter

- ½ Vidalia onion, thinly sliced

- 1 cup low-sodium vegetable broth

- 3 cups fresh shelled peas

- 1 tablespoon minced fresh tarragon

Melt the butter in a skillet over medium heat.

Sauté the onion in the melted butter for about 3 minutes until translucent, stirring occasionally.

Pour in the vegetable broth and whisk well. Add the peas and tarragon to the skillet and stir to combine.

Reduce the heat to low, cover, and cook for about 8 minutes more, or until the peas are tender.

Let the peas cool for 5 minutes and serve warm.

Nutritional Info:

calories: 82 | fat: 2.1g | protein: 4.2g | carbs: 12.0g | fiber: 3.8g | sugar: 4.9g | sodium: 48mg

Grilled Zucchini With Tomato Relish

Servings: 4

Cooking Time: 10 Minutes

Ingredients:

- 1 lb. zucchini, sliced in half

- 1 tablespoon olive oil

- Salt and pepper to taste

- 1 teaspoon red wine vinegar

- 1 tablespoon mint, chopped

- 1 cup tomatoes, chopped

Directions:

Preheat your grill.

Brush both sides of zucchini with oil and season with salt and pepper.

Grill for 3 to 4 minutes per side.

In a bowl, mix the rest of the ingredients with the remaining oil.

Season with salt and pepper.

Spread tomato relish on top of the grilled zucchini before serving.

Nutrition Info:

Calories 71 Total Fat 5 g Saturated Fat 1 g Cholesterol 0 mg Sodium 157 mg Total Carbohydrate 6 g Dietary Fiber 2 g Total Sugars 4 g Protein 2 g Potassium 413 mg

Pickled Cucumbers

Preparation Time: 15 minutes | Cooking Time: 5 minutes | Servings: 10

- 2 cucumbers, cut into ¼-inch slices
- ½ onion, sliced thin
- 1½ cups vinegar
- 2 tablespoons stevia
- 1 tablespoon dill
- 2 cloves garlic, sliced thin
- 1 teaspoon peppercorns
- 1 teaspoon coriander seeds
- ½ teaspoon salt
- ¼ teaspoon red pepper flakes

In a medium saucepan, combine vinegar and spices. Bring to a boil over high heat. Set aside.

Place the cucumbers, onions, and garlic into a quart-sized jar, or plastic container, with an air tight lid. Pour hot liquid over the vegetables, making sure they are completely covered.

Add the lid and chill at least a day before serving.

Nutritional Info:

calories: 35 | fat: 0g | protein: 0g | carbs: 6.1g | fiber: 0g | sugar: 4.0g | sodium: 124mg

Lemony Brussels Sprouts

Preparation Time: 10 minutes | Cooking Time: 20 minutes | Servings: 4

- 1 pound (454 g) Brussels sprouts
- 2 tablespoons avocado oil, divided
- 1 cup vegetable broth or chicken bone broth
- 1 tablespoon minced garlic
- ½ teaspoon kosher salt
- Freshly ground black pepper, to taste
- ½ medium lemon
- ½ tablespoon poppy seeds

Trim the Brussels sprouts by cutting off the stem ends and removing any loose outer leaves. Cut each in half lengthwise (through the stem).

Set the electric pressure cooker to the Sauté/More setting. When the pot is hot, pour in 1 tablespoon of the avocado oil.

Add half of the Brussels sprouts to the pot, cut-side down, and let them brown for 3 to 5 minutes without disturbing. Transfer to a bowl and add the remaining tablespoon of avocado oil and the remaining Brussels sprouts to the pot. Hit Cancel and return all of the Brussels sprouts to the pot.

Add the broth, garlic, salt, and a few grinds of pepper. Stir to distribute the seasonings.

Close and lock the lid of the pressure cooker. Set the valve to sealing.

Cook on high pressure for 2 minutes.

While the Brussels sprouts are cooking, zest the lemon, then cut it into quarters.

When the cooking is complete, hit Cancel and quick release the pressure.

Once the pin drops, unlock and remove the lid.

Using a slotted spoon, transfer the Brussels sprouts to a serving bowl. Toss with the lemon zest, a squeeze of lemon juice, and the poppy seeds. Serve immediately.

Nutritional Info:

calories: 126 | fat: 8.1g | protein: 4.1g | carbs: 12.9g | fiber: 4.9g | sugar: 3.0g | sodium: 500mg

Mushroom Toast

Servings: 8

Cooking Time: 10 Minutes

Ingredients:

- 1 lb. button mushrooms

- 2 tablespoons thyme, chopped

- 3 tablespoons parsley, chopped

- 2 celery stalks, chopped

- 8 whole-grain bread slices, 1-inch slices

- What you will need from the store cupboard:

- 2 tablespoons sour cream, low-fat

- 1 crushed garlic clove

- ½ cup ricotta cheese

- Pinch of cayenne pepper

- Salt and pepper to taste

Directions:

Keep the celery, ricotta, cayenne pepper and parsley in a bowl. Mix well.

Preheat your oven to 350 °F.

Halve the large mushrooms. Place them in a big skillet.

Add the thyme, garlic, sour cream, and 1 teaspoon of water.

Cook covered until your mushrooms have become tender.

Season with pepper and salt.

In the meantime, toast both sides of the bread slices.

Apply ricotta mixture on one side of the toast. Cut it in half.

Place toasts on serving plates.

Now spoon the mushroom mixture over them before serving.

Nutrition Info:

Calories 148, Carbohydrates 24g, Fiber 4g, Cholesterol 6mg, Sugar 0.3g, Fat 4g, Protein 8g

Butternut Fritters

Servings: 6

Cooking Time: 15 Minutes

Ingredients:

- 5 cup butternut squash, grated

- 2 large eggs

- 1 tablespoon. fresh sage, diced fine

- 2/3 cup flour

- 2 tablespoons olive oil

- Salt and pepper, to taste

Directions:

Heat oil in a large skillet over med-high heat.

In a large bowl, combine squash, eggs, sage and salt and pepper to taste. Fold in flour.

Drop ¼ cup mixture into skillet, keeping fritters at least 1 inch apart. Cook till golden brown on both sides, about 2 minutes per side.

Transfer to paper towel lined plate. Repeat. Serve immediately with your favorite dipping sauce.

Nutrition Info:

Calories 164 Total Carbohydrates 24g Net Carbohydrates 21g Protein 4g Fat 6g Sugar 3g Fiber 3g

Cauliflower In Vegan Alfredo Sauce

Servings: 1

Cooking Time: 35 Minutes

Ingredients:

- Olive oil: 1 tablespoon

- Garlic: 2 cloves

- Vegetable broth: 1 cup

- Sea salt: ½ teaspoon

- Pepper: as per taste

- Chilli flakes: 1 teaspoon

- Onion (diced): 1 medium

- Cauliflower florets (chopped): 4 cups

- Lemon juice (freshly squeezed): 1 teaspoon

- nutritional yeast: 1 tablespoon

- Vegan butter: 2 tablespoons

- Zucchini noodles: for serving

Directions:

Begin by positioning a cooking pot on low heat. Stream in the oil and allow it to heat through.

Immediately you're done, toss in the chopped onion and set on fire for about 4 minutes. The onion should be translucent.

Put in the garlic and Prepare for about 30 seconds. Continuously stir to prevent them from sticking.

Put in the vegetable broth and shredded cauliflower florets. Ensure you mix well and cover the stockpot with a lid. Allow the cauliflower cook for 5 minutes and then extract it from the flame.

Get a blender and move the cooked cauliflower into it. Palpitate until the puree is smooth and creamy in texture. (Add 1 tablespoon of broth if required for.)

Put salt, lemon juice, nutritional yeast, butter, chilli flakes, and pepper to the blender. Mix until all the ingredients fully combine to form a smooth puree.

Position the zucchini noodles over a dishing platter and stream the Prepare cauliflower Alfredo sauce over the noodles.

Nutrition Info:

Fat: 9.1 g Protein: 3.9 g Carbohydrates: 10 g

Tempeh With Bell Peppers

Servings: 3

Cooking Time: 15 Minutes

Ingredients:

- 2 tablespoons balsamic vinegar

- 2 tablespoons low-sodium soy sauce

- 2 tablespoons tomato sauce

- 1 teaspoon maple syrup

- ½ teaspoon garlic powder

- 1/8 teaspoon red pepper flakes, crushed

- 1 tablespoon vegetable oil

- 8 ounces' tempeh, cut into cubes

- 1 medium onion, chopped

- 2 large green bell peppers, seeded and chopped

Directions:

In a small bowl, add the vinegar, soy sauce, tomato sauce, maple syrup, garlic powder, and red pepper flakes and beat until well combined. Set aside.

Heat 1 tablespoon of oil in a large skillet over medium heat and cook the tempeh about 2–3 minutes per side.

Add the onion and bell peppers and heat for about 2–3 minutes.

Stir in the sauce mixture and cook for about 3–5 minutes, stirring frequently.

Serve hot.

Nutrition Info:

Calories 241 Total Fat 13 g

Saturated Fat 2.6 g

Cholesterol 0 mg Sodium 65 mg

Total Carbs 19.7 g Fiber 2.1 g

Sugar 8.1 g Protein 16.1 g

Broccoli With Ginger And Garlic

Servings: 4

Cooking Time: 11 Minutes

Ingredients:

- 2 tablespoons extra-virgin olive oil

- 2 cups broccoli florets

- 1 tablespoon grated fresh ginger

- ½ teaspoon sea salt

- ⅛ teaspoon freshly ground black pepper

- 3 garlic cloves, minced

Directions:

In a large skillet over medium-high heat, heat the olive oil until it shimmers.

Add the broccoli, ginger, sea salt, and pepper. Cook for about 10 minutes, stirring occasionally, until the broccoli is soft and starts to brown.

Add the garlic and cook for 30 seconds, stirring constantly. Remove from the heat and serve.

Nutrition Info:

Per Serving Calories: 80; Protein: 1g; Total Carbohydrates: 4g; Sugars: 1g; Fiber: 1g; Total Fat: 0g; Saturated Fat: 1g; Cholesterol: 0mg; Sodium: 249mg

Carrot Soup With Tempeh

Servings: 6

Cooking Time: 45 Minutes

Ingredients:

- ¼ cup olive oil, divided
- 1 large yellow onion, chopped
- Salt, to taste
- 2 pounds' carrots, peeled, and cut into ½-inch rounds
- 2 tablespoons fresh dill, chopped
- 4½ cups homemade vegetable broth
- 12 ounces' tempeh, cut into ½-inch cubes
- ¼ cup tomato paste
- 1 teaspoon fresh lemon juice

Directions:

In a large soup pan, heat 2 tablespoons of the oil over medium heat and cook the onion with salt for about 6–8 minutes, stirring frequently.

Add the carrots and stir to combine.

Lower the heat to low and cook, covered for about 5 minutes, stirring frequently.

Add in the broth and bring to a boil over high heat.

Lower the heat to a low and simmer, covered for about 30 minutes.

Meanwhile, in a skillet, heat the remaining oil over medium-high heat and cook the tempeh for about 3–5 minutes.

Stir in the dill and cook for about 1 minute.

Remove from the heat.

Remove the pan of soup from heat and stir in tomato paste and lemon juice.

With an immersion blender, blend the soup until smooth and creamy.

Serve the soup hot with the topping of tempeh.

Nutrition Info:

Calories 294 Total Fat 15.7 g Saturated Fat 2.8 g Cholesterol 0 mg Sodium 723 mg Total Carbs 25.9 g Fiber 4.9 g Sugar 10.4 g Protein 16.4 g

Jicama with Guacamole

Preparation Time: 5 minutes | Cooking Time: 0 minutes | Servings: 4

- 1 avocado, cut into cubes

- Juice of ½ lime

- 2 tablespoons finely chopped red onion

- 2 tablespoons chopped fresh cilantro

- 1 garlic clove, minced

- ¼ teaspoon sea salt

- 1 cup sliced jicama

In a small bowl, combine the avocado, lime juice, onion, cilantro, garlic, and salt. Mash lightly with a fork.

Serve with the jicama for dipping.

Nutritional Info:

calories: 74 | fat: 5.1g | protein: 1.1g | carbs: 7.9g | fiber: 4.9g | sugar: 3.0g | sodium: 80mg

Peppers with Zucchini Dip

Preparation Time: 10 minutes | Cooking Time: 0 minutes | Servings: 4

- 2 zucchini, chopped

- 3 garlic cloves

- 2 tablespoons extra-virgin olive oil

- 2 tablespoons tahini

- Juice of 1 lemon

- ½ teaspoon sea salt

- 1 red bell pepper, seeded and cut into sticks

In a blender or food processor, combine the zucchini, garlic, olive oil, tahini, lemon juice, and salt. Blend until smooth.

Serve with the red bell pepper for dipping.

Nutritional Info:

calories: 120 | fat: 11.1g | protein: 2.1g | carbs: 6.9g | fiber: 2.9g | sugar: 4.0g | sodium: 155mg

Beans, Walnuts & Veggie Burgers

Servings: 8

Cooking Time: 25 Minutes

Ingredients:

- ½ cup walnuts
- 1 carrot, peeled and chopped
- 1 celery stalk, chopped
- 4 scallions, chopped
- 5 garlic cloves, chopped
- 2¼ cups cooked black beans
- 2½ cups sweet potato, peeled and grated
- ½ teaspoon red pepper flakes, crushed
- ¼ teaspoon cayenne pepper
- Salt and ground black pepper, as required

Directions:

Preheat the oven to 400 degrees F. Line a baking sheet with parchment paper.

In a food processor, add walnuts and pulse until finely ground.

Add the carrot, celery, scallion and garlic and pulse until chopped finely.

Transfer the vegetable mixture into a large bowl.

In the same food processor, add beans and pulse until chopped.

Add 1½ cups of sweet potato and pulse until a chunky mixture forms.

Transfer the bean mixture into the bowl with vegetable mixture.

Stir in the remaining sweet potato and spices and mix until well combined.

Make 8 patties from mixture.

Arrange the patties onto prepared baking sheet in a single layer.

Bake for about 25 minutes.

Serve hot.

Meal Prep Tip: Remove the burgers from oven and set aside to cool completely. Store these burgers in an airtight container, by placing parchment papers between the burgers to avoid the sticking. These burgers can be stored in the freezer for up to 3 weeks. Before serving, thaw the burgers and then reheat in microwave.

Nutrition Info:

Calories 177 Total Fat 5 g Saturated Fat 0.3 g Cholesterol 0 mg Total Carbs 27.6 g Sugar 5.3 g Fiber 7.6 g Sodium 205 mg Potassium 398 mg Protein 8 g

Balsamic Roasted Carrots

Servings: 4

Cooking Time: 30 Minutes

Ingredients:

- 1½ pounds carrots, quartered lengthwise
- 2 tablespoons extra-virgin olive oil
- ¼ teaspoon sea salt
- ⅛ teaspoon freshly ground black pepper
- 3 tablespoons balsamic vinegar

Directions:

Preheat the oven to 425°F.

In a large bowl, toss the carrots with the olive oil, sea salt, and pepper. Place in a single layer in a roasting pan or on a rimmed baking sheet. Roast for 20 to 30 minutes until the carrots are caramelized.

Toss with the vinegar and serve.

Nutrition Info:

Calories: 132; Protein: 1g; Total Carbohydrates: 17g

Sugars: 8g; Fiber: 4g; Total Fat: 7g; Saturated Fat: 1g

Cholesterol: 0mg; Sodium: 235mg

Roasted Asparagus and Red Peppers

Preparation Time: 5 minutes | Cooking Time: 15 minutes | Servings: 4

- 1 pound (454 g) asparagus, woody ends trimmed, cut into 2-inch segments

- 2 red bell peppers, seeded, cut into 1-inch pieces

- 1 small onion, quartered

- 2 tablespoons Italian dressing

Preheat the oven to 400°F (205°C). Line a baking sheet with parchment paper and set aside.

Combine the asparagus with the peppers, onion, and dressing in a large bowl, and toss well.

Arrange the vegetables on the baking sheet and roast for about 15 minutes until softened. Flip the vegetables with a spatula once during cooking.

Transfer to a large platter and serve.

Nutritional Info:

calories: 92 | fat: 4.8g | protein: 2.9g | carbs: 10.7g | fiber: 4.0g | sugar: 5.7g | sodium: 31mg

Boiled Potatoes With Tomato Salsa

Servings: 8

Cooking Time: 15 Minutes

Ingredients:

- 6 potatoes, sliced into wedges

- 1 clove garlic, minced

- 3 large tomatoes, diced

- 2 tablespoons white onion, chopped

- 2 teaspoons fresh marjoram, chopped

- Salt and pepper to taste

Directions:

Boil the potatoes until soft enough to poke with a fork.

Combine the rest of the ingredients in a bowl.

Serve potatoes with salsa.

Nutrition Info:

Calories 200 Total Fat 10 g Saturated Fat 1 g

Cholesterol 25 mg Sodium 81 mg Total

Carbohydrate 10 g Dietary Fiber 5 g Total

Sugars 1 g Protein 25 g Potassium 560 mg

Bean Medley Chili

Servings: 8

Cooking Time: 20 Minutes

Ingredients:

- 1 can black beans, rinsed and drained

- 1 can garbanzo beans, rinsed and drained

- 1 teaspoon cumin, ground

- ¼ cup cilantro, snipped

- 2 onions, chopped

- What you will need from the store cupboard:

- 1 can chicken broth

- 3 tablespoons of chili powder

- 1 can chipotle chili pepper in adobo sauce

- ¼ teaspoon salt

Directions:

Bring together the beans, pepper, onion, chili powder, salt, and cumin in your cooker.

Add the broth.

Cover and cook.

Stir the cilantro in.

You can serve it with rice if desired.

Nutrition Info:

Calories 191

Carbohydrates 38g

Cholesterol 0mg

Fiber 12g, Fat 2g

Protein 12g

Sugar 0.7g

Sodium 659mg

Barley Pilaf

Servings: 4

Cooking Time: 1 Hour 5 Minutes

Ingredients:

- ½ cup pearl barley

- 1 cup low-sodium vegetable broth

- 2 tablespoons olive oil, divided

- 2 garlic cloves, minced finely

- ½ cup onion, chopped

- ½ cup eggplant, sliced thinly

- ½ cup green bell pepper, seeded and chopped

- ½ cup red bell pepper, seeded and chopped

- 2 tablespoons fresh cilantro, chopped

- 2 tablespoons fresh mint leaves, chopped

Directions:

In a pan, add the barley and broth over medium-high heat and bring to a boil.

Immediately, reduce the heat to low and simmer, covered for about 45 minutes or until all the liquid is absorbed.

In a large skillet, heat 1 tablespoon of oil over high heat and sauté the garlic for about 1 minute.

Stir in the cooked barley and cook for about 3 minutes.

Remove from heat and set aside.

In another skillet, heat remaining oil over medium heat and sauté the onion for about 5-7 minutes.

Add the eggplant and bell peppers and stir fry for about 3 minutes.

Stir in the remaining ingredients except walnuts and cook for about 2-3 minutes.

Stir in barley mixture and cook for about 2-3 minutes.

Serve hot.

Meal Prep Tip: Transfer the pilaf into a large bowl and set aside to cool. Divide the pilaf into 4 containers evenly. Cover the containers and refrigerate for 1 day. Reheat in the microwave before serving.

Nutrition Info:

Calories 168 Total Fat 7.4 g Saturated Fat 1.1 g Cholesterol 0 mg Total Carbs 23.5 g Sugar 1.9 g Fiber 5 g Sodium 22 mg Potassium 164 mg Protein 3.6 g

Asian Fried Eggplant

Servings: 4

Cooking Time: 40 Minutes

Ingredients:

- 1 large eggplant, sliced into fourths

- 3 green onions, diced, green tips only

- 1 teaspoon fresh ginger, peeled & diced fine

- ¼ cup + 1 teaspoon cornstarch

- 1 ½ tablespoon. soy sauce

- 1 ½ tablespoon. sesame oil

- 1 tablespoon. vegetable oil

- 1 tablespoon. fish sauce

- 2 teaspoon Splenda

- ¼ teaspoon salt

Directions:

Place eggplant on paper towels and sprinkle both sides with salt. Let for 1 hour to remove excess moisture. Pat dry with more paper towels.

In a small bowl, whisk together soy sauce, sesame oil, fish sauce, Splenda, and 1 teaspoon cornstarch.

Coat both sides of the eggplant with the ¼ cup cornstarch, use more if needed.

Heat oil in a large skillet, over med-high heat. Add ½ the ginger and 1 green onion, then lay 2 slices of eggplant on top. Use ½ the sauce mixture to lightly coat both sides of the eggplant. Cook 8-10 minutes per side. Repeat.

Serve garnished with remaining green onions.

Nutrition Info:

Calories 155 Total

Carbohydrates 18g

Net Carbohydrates 13g

Protein 2g

Fat 9g

Sugar 6g

Fiber 5g

Cucumber Salad With Pesto

Servings: 4

Cooking Time: 0 Minute

Ingredients:

- 1 cup fresh basil leaves, chopped

- 2 cloves garlic

- 2 tablespoons walnuts

- 1 teaspoon Parmesan cheese

- 1 tablespoon olive oil

- 2 cucumbers, sliced into rounds

- Salt and pepper to taste

Directions:

Put the basil, garlic, walnuts, Parmesan cheese and olive oil in a food processor.

Pulse until smooth.

Season the cucumbers with salt and pepper.

Spread pesto on top of each cucumber round.

Nutrition Info:

Calories 80 Total Fat 6g Saturated Fat 0.7g Cholesterol 0mg Sodium 4mg Total Carbohydrate 6.5g Dietary Fiber 1.2g Total Sugars 2.6g Protein 2.2g Potassium 266mg

Roasted Carrots

Servings: 4

Cooking Time: 20 Minutes

Ingredients:

- 2 tablespoons olive oil, divided

- 2 tablespoons balsamic vinegar

- 1 tablespoon pure maple syrup

- 1 lb. carrots, sliced into small pieces

- Salt to taste

- 2 tablespoons hazelnuts, chopped

Directions:

Preheat your oven to 400 degrees F.

Combine 1 tablespoon oil with vinegar and maple syrup.

Set aside the mixture.

In another bowl, toss the carrots in remaining oil and season with salt.

Arrange on a single layer in a baking pan.

Roast for 15 minutes.

Pour the reserved mixture over the carrots and mix.

Roast for additional 5 minutes.

Sprinkle hazelnuts on top before serving.

Nutrition Info:

Calories 130

Total Fat 7 g

Saturated Fat 1g

Cholesterol 0 mg

Sodium 226 mg

Total Carbohydrate 16 g

Dietary Fiber 3 g

Total Sugars 10 g

Protein 1 g

Potassium 382 mg

Kale With Miso & Ginger

Servings: 6

Cooking Time: 10 Minutes

Ingredients:

- 8 oz. fresh kale, sliced into strips

- 1 clove garlic, minced

- 1 tablespoon lime juice

- ½ teaspoon lime zest

- 2 tablespoons oil

- 2 tablespoons rice vinegar

- 1 teaspoon fresh ginger, grated

- 2 teaspoons miso

- 2 tablespoons dry roasted cashews, chopped

Directions:

Steam kale on a steamer basket in a pot with water.

Transfer kale to a bowl.

Mix the rest of the ingredients except cashews in another bowl.

Toss kale in the mixture.

Top with chopped cashews before serving.

Nutrition Info:

Calories 86 Total

Fat 5 g

Saturated Fat 0 g

Cholesterol 0 mg

Sodium 104 mg

Total Carbohydrate 9 g

Dietary Fiber 2 g

Total Sugars 2 g

Protein 3 g

Potassium 352 mg

Beet Soup

Servings: 2

Cooking Time: 5 Minutes

Ingredients:

- 2 cups coconut yogurt
- 4 teaspoons fresh lemon juice
- 2 cups beets, trimmed, peeled, and chopped
- 2 tablespoons fresh dill
- Salt, to taste
- 1 tablespoon pumpkin seeds
- 2 tablespoons coconut cream
- 1 tablespoon fresh chives, minced

Directions:

In a high-speed blender, add all ingredients and pulse until smooth.

Transfer the soup into a pan over medium heat and cook for about 3–5 minutes or until heated through.

Serve immediately with the garnishing of chives and coconut cream.

Nutrition Info:

Calories 230 Total Fat 8 g Saturated Fat 5.8 g Cholesterol 0 mg Sodium 218 mg Total Carbs 33.5 g Fiber 4.2 g Sugar 27.5 g Protein 8 g

Quinoa In Tomato Sauce

Servings: 4

Cooking Time: 40 Minutes

Ingredients:

- 2 tablespoons olive oil

- 1 cup quinoa, rinsed

- 1 green bell pepper, seeded and chopped

- 1 medium onion, chopped finely

- 3 garlic cloves, minced

- 2½ cups filtered water

- 2 cups tomatoes, crushed finely

- 1 teaspoon red chili powder

- ¼ teaspoon ground cumin

- ¼ teaspoon garlic powder

- Ground black pepper, as required

Directions:

In a large pan, heat the oil over medium-high heat and cook the quinoa, onion, bell pepper and garlic for about 5 minutes, stirring frequently.

Stir in the remaining ingredients and bring to a boil.

Now, reduce the heat to medium-low.

Cover the pan tightly and simmer for about 3o minutes, stirring occasionally.

Serve hot.

Meal Prep Tip: Transfer the quinoa mixture into a large bowl and set aside to cool. Divide the chili into 4 containers evenly. Cover the containers and refrigerate for 1-2 days. Reheat in the microwave before serving.

Nutrition Info:

Calories 260 Total Fat 10 g Saturated Fat 1.4 g Cholesterol 0 mg Total Carbs 36.9 g Sugar 5.2 g Fiber 5.4 g Sodium 16 mg Potassium 575 mg Protein 7.7 g

Cauliflower Mushroom Risotto

Servings: 2

Cooking Time: 30 Minutes

Ingredients:

- 1 medium head cauliflower, grated

- 8-ounce Porcini mushrooms, sliced

- 1 yellow onion, diced fine

- 2 cup low sodium vegetable broth

- 2 teaspoon garlic, diced fine

- 2 teaspoon white wine vinegar

- Salt & pepper, to taste

- Olive oil cooking spray

Directions:

Heat oven to 350 degrees. Line a baking sheet with foil.

Place the mushrooms on the prepared pan and spray with cooking spray. Sprinkle with salt and toss to coat. Bake 10-12 minutes, or until golden brown and the mushrooms start to crisp.

Spray a large skillet with cooking spray and place over med-high heat. Add onion and cook, stirring frequently, until translucent, about 3-4 minutes. Add garlic and cook 2 minutes, until golden.

Add the cauliflower and cook 1 minute, stirring.

Place the broth in a saucepan and bring to a simmer. Add to the skillet, ¼ cup at a time, mixing well after each addition.

Stir in vinegar. Reduce heat to low and let simmer, 4-5 minutes, or until most of the liquid has evaporated.

Spoon cauliflower mixture onto plates, or in bowls, and top with mushrooms. Serve.

Nutrition Info:

Calories 134 Total

Carbohydrates 22g

Protein 10g

Fat 0g

Sugar 5g

Fiber 2g

Mushroom Curry

Servings: 3

Cooking Time: 20 Minutes

Ingredients:

- 2 cups tomatoes, chopped

- 1 green chili, chopped

- 1 teaspoon fresh ginger, chopped

- ¼ cup cashews

- 2 tablespoons canola oil

- ½ teaspoon cumin seeds

- ¼ teaspoon ground coriander

- ¼ teaspoon ground turmeric

- ¼ teaspoon red chili powder

- 1½ cups fresh shiitake mushrooms, sliced

- 1½ cups fresh button mushrooms, sliced

- 1 cup frozen corn kernels

- 1¼ cups water

- ¼ cup unsweetened coconut milk

- Salt and ground black pepper, to taste

Directions:

In a food processor, add the tomatoes, green chili, ginger, and cashews, and pulse until a smooth paste forms.

In a pan, heat the oil over medium heat and sauté the cumin seeds for about 1 minute.

Add the spices and sauté for about 1 minute.

Add the tomato paste and cook for about 5 minutes.

Stir in the mushrooms, corn, water, and coconut milk, and bring to a boil.

Cook for about 10–12 minutes, stirring occasionally.

Season with salt and black pepper and remove from the heat.

Serve hot.

Nutrition Info:

Calories 311 Total Fat 20.4 g Saturated Fat 6.1 g Cholesterol 0 mg Sodium 244 mg Total Carbs 32g Fiber 5.6 g Sugar 9 g Protein 8 g

Squash Medley

Servings: 2

Cooking Time: 20 Minutes.

Ingredients:

- 2lbs mixed squash
- 0.5 cup mixed veg
- 1 cup vegetable stock
- 2tbsp olive oil
- 2tbsp mixed herbs

Directions:

Put the squash in the steamer basket and add the stock into the Instant Pot.

Steam the squash in your Instant Pot for 10 minutes.

Depressurize and pour away the remaining stock.

Set to saute and add the oil and remaining ingredients.

Cook until a light crust forms.

Nutrition Info:

Calories: 100 Carbs: 10 Sugar: 3 Fat: 6 Protein: 5 GL: 20

Banana Curry

Servings: 3

Cooking Time: 15 Minutes

Ingredients:

- 2 tablespoons olive

- 2 yellow onions, chopped

- 8 garlic cloves, minced

- 2 tablespoons curry powder

- 1 tablespoon ground ginger

- 1 tablespoon ground cumin

- 1 teaspoon ground turmeric

- 1 teaspoon ground cinnamon

- 1 teaspoon red chili powder

- Salt and ground black pepper, to taste

- 2/3 cup soy yogurt

- 1 cup tomato puree

- 2 bananas, peeled and sliced

- 3 tomatoes, chopped finely

- ¼ cup unsweetened coconut flakes

Directions:

In a large pan, heat the oil over medium heat and sauté onion for about 4–5 minutes.

Add the garlic, curry powder, and spices, and sauté for about 1 minute.

Add the soy yogurt and tomato sauce and bring to a gentle boil.

Stir in the bananas and simmer for about 3 minutes.

Stir in the tomatoes and simmer for about 1–2 minutes.

Stir in the coconut flakes and immediately remove from the heat.

Serve hot.

Nutrition Info:

Calories 382 Total Fat 18.2 g

Saturated Fat 6.6 g

Cholesterol 0 mg Sodium 108 mg

Total Carbs 53.4 g Fiber 11.3 g

Sugar 24.8 g Protein 9 g

Tofu Curry

Servings: 2

Cooking Time: 20 Minutes

Ingredients:

- 2 cups cubed extra firm tofu
- 2 cups mixed stir fry vegetables
- 0.5 cup soy yogurt
- 3tbsp curry paste
- 1tbsp oil or ghee

Directions:

Set the Instant Pot to saute and add the oil and curry paste.

When the onion is soft, add the remaining ingredients except the yogurt and seal.

Cook on Stew for 20 minutes.

Release the pressure naturally and serve with a scoop of soy yogurt.

Nutrition Info:

Calories: 300 Carbs: 9 Sugar: 4 Fat: 14 Protein: 42 GL: 7

Roasted Lemon Mixed Vegetables

Servings: 5

Cooking Time: 20 Minutes

Ingredients:

- 2 teaspoons lemon zest

- 1-1/2 cups broccoli florets

- 1-1/2 cups cauliflower florets

- 1 teaspoon oregano, crushed

- ¾ cup red bell pepper, diced

- What you will need from the store cupboard:

- 1 tablespoon olive oil

- 2 sliced garlic cloves

- ¼ teaspoon salt

Directions:

Preheat your oven to 350 °F.

Bring together the broccoli, garlic, and cauliflower in a baking pan.

Drizzle oil. Sprinkle the salt and oregano.

Roast for 10 minutes.

Now add the bell pepper to the vegetables. Stir and combine.

Roast until the vegetables have become light brown and crisp.

Sprinkle lemon zest and serve.

Nutrition Info:

Calories 52

Carbohydrates 5g

Fiber 2g

Cholesterol 0mg

Fat 3g

Sugar 0.2g

Protein 2g

Sodium 134mg

Mixed Greens Salad

Servings: 6

Cooking Time: 0 Minutes

Ingredients:

- 6 cups mixed salad greens

- 1 cup cucumber, chopped

- ½ cup carrot, shredded

- ¼ cup bell pepper, sliced into strips

- ¼ cup cherry tomatoes, sliced in half

- 6 tablespoons white onion, chopped

- 6 tablespoons balsamic vinaigrette dressing

Directions:

Toss all the ingredients in a large salad bowl.

Drizzle dressing on top or serve on the side.

Nutrition Info:

Calories 23 Total Fat 1 g Saturated Fat 0 g Cholesterol 0 mg Sodium 138 mg Total Carbohydrate 4 g Dietary Fiber 1 g Total Sugars 1 g Protein 1 g Potassium 142 mg

Spicy Black Beans

Servings: 6

Cooking Time: 1½ Hours

Ingredients:

- 4 cups filtered water

- 1½ cups dried black beans, soaked for 8 hours and drained

- ½ teaspoon ground turmeric

- 3 tablespoons olive oil

- 1 small onion, chopped finely

- 1 green chili, chopped

- 1 (1-inch) piece fresh ginger, minced

- 2 garlic cloves, minced

- 1-1½ tablespoons ground coriander

- 1 teaspoon ground cumin

- ½ teaspoon cayenne pepper

- Sea salt, as required

- 2 medium tomatoes, chopped finely

- ½ cup fresh cilantro, chopped

Directions:

In a large pan, add water, black beans and turmeric and bring to a boil on high heat.

Now, reduce the heat to low and simmer, covered for about 1 hour or till desired doneness of beans.

Meanwhile, in a skillet, heat the oil over medium heat and sauté the onion for about 4-5 minutes.

Add the green chili, ginger, garlic, spices and salt and sauté for about 1-2 minutes.

Stir in the tomatoes and cook for about 10 minutes, stirring occasionally.

Transfer the tomato mixture into the pan with black beans and stir to combine.

Increase the heat to medium-low and simmer for about 15-20 minutes.

Stir in the cilantro and simmer for about 5 minutes.

Serve hot.

Meal Prep Tip: Transfer the beans mixture into a large bowl and set aside to cool. Divide the mixture into 6 containers evenly. Cover the containers and refrigerate for 1-2 days. Reheat in the microwave before serving.

Nutrition Info:

Calories 160 Total Fat 8 g Saturated Fat 1 g Cholesterol 0 mg Total Carbs 17.9 g Sugar 2.4 g Fiber 6.2 g Sodium 50 mg Potassium 343 mg Protein 6 g

Mini Eggplant Pizzas

Preparation Time: 15 minutes | Cooking Time: 1 hour 10 minutes | Servings: 4

- 1 large eggplant, peeled and sliced into ¼-inch circles

- ½ cup reduced-fat Mozzarella cheese, grated

- 2 eggs

- 1¼ cups Italian bread crumbs

- 1 tablespoon water

- ¼ teaspoon black pepper

- Nonstick cooking spray

Spaghetti Sauce:

- 1 onion, diced

- 1 carrot, grated

- 1 stalk celery, diced

- 1 zucchini, grated

- 1 (28-ounce / 794-g) Italian-style tomatoes, in puree

- 1 (14½-ounce / 411-g) diced tomatoes, with juice

- ½ cup water

- 2 cloves garlic, diced fine

- ½ tablespoon oregano

- 1 teaspoon olive oil

- 1 teaspoon basil

- 1 teaspoon thyme

- 1 teaspoon salt

- ¼ teaspoon red pepper flakes

Heat oven to 350°F (180°C). Line 2 large cookie sheets with foil and spray well with cooking spray.

In a shallow dish, beat eggs, water and pepper. Place the bread crumbs in a separate shallow dish.

Dip eggplant pieces in egg mixture, then coat completely with bread crumbs. Place on prepared cookie sheets. Spray the tops with cooking spray and bake 15 minutes.

Turn the eggplant over and spray with cooking spray again. Bake another 15 minutes.

Meanwhile, make the spaghetti sauce: Heat oil in a large saucepan over medium heat. Add vegetables and garlic. Cook, stirring frequently, until vegetables get soft, about 5 minutes.

Add remaining Ingredients, use the back of a spoon to break up tomatoes.

Bring to a simmer and cook, partially covered, over medium-low heat 30 minutes, stirring frequently.

Remove the eggplant from oven and top each piece with 1 tablespoon spaghetti sauce. Sprinkle cheese over sauce and bake for another 4 to 5 minutes, or until sauce is bubbly and cheese is melted.

Serve immediately.

Nutritional Info:

calories: 172 | fat: 5.0g | protein: 9.2g | carbs: 24.1g | fiber: 4.0g | sugar: 6.0g | sodium: 1005mg

Baked Beans

Servings: 6

Cooking Time: 20 Minutes

Ingredients:

- 2 cups navy beans, overnight soaked in cold water

- 2/3 cups green bell pepper, diced

- 1 can tomatoes, diced

- 1 onion, sliced

- What you will need from the store cupboard:

- 3 tablespoons molasses

- ¼ cup of orange juice

- ¼ cup maple syrup

- 1 tablespoon Worcestershire sauce

- 1/4 teaspoon mustard powder

- 2 tablespoons stevia sugar

- 2 tablespoons salt

Directions:

Preheat your oven to 350 °F

Simmer the beans. Drain and keep the liquid.

Place beans in a casserole dish with the onion.

Bring together the dry mustard, pepper, salt, molasses, Worcestershire sauce, tomatoes, sugar substitute and orange juice in your saucepan.

Boil the mix. Pour over your beans.

Pour the reserved bean water, covering the beans.

Use aluminum foil to cover the dish.

Now bake in the oven. The beans must get tender.

Remove the foil and add some liquid if needed.

Nutrition Info:

Calories 482, Carbohydrates 65g, Cholesterol 25mg, Fiber 12g, Fat 16g, Protein 21g, Sugar 2.2g, Sodium 512mg

Lentil And Eggplant Stew

Servings: 2

Cooking Time: 35 Minutes

Ingredients:

- 1lb eggplant

- 1lb dry lentils

- 1 cup chopped vegetables

- 1 cup low sodium vegetable broth

Directions:

Mix all the ingredients in your Instant Pot.

Cook on Stew for 35 minutes.

Release the pressure naturally.

Nutrition Info:

Calories: 310

Carbs: 22

Sugar: 6

Fat: 10

Protein: 32 GL: 16

Butter-Orange Yams

Preparation Time: 7 minutes | Cooking Time: 45 minutes | Servings: 8 (½ cup each)

- 2 medium jewel yams, cut into 2-inch dices

- 2 tablespoons unsalted butter

- Juice of 1 large orange

- 1½ teaspoons ground cinnamon

- ¼ teaspoon ground ginger

- ¾ teaspoon ground nutmeg

- ⅛ teaspoon ground cloves

Preheat the oven to 350°F (180°C).

Arrange the yam dices on a rimmed baking sheet in a single layer. Set aside.

Add the butter, orange juice, cinnamon, ginger, nutmeg, and garlic cloves to a medium saucepan over medium-low heat. Cook for 3 to 5 minutes, stirring continuously, or until the sauce begins to thicken and bubble.

Spoon the sauce over the yams and toss to coat well.

Bake in the preheated oven for 40 minutes until tender.

Let the yams cool for 8 minutes in the baking sheet before removing and serving.

Nutritional Info:

Calories: 129 | fat: 2.8g

Protein: 2.1g | carbs: 24.7g

Fiber: 5.0g | sugar: 2.9g

Sodium: 28mg

Tofu With Peas

Servings: 5

Cooking Time: 20 Minutes

Ingredients:

- 1 tablespoon chili-garlic sauce

- 3 tablespoons low-sodium soy sauce

- 2 tablespoons canola oil, divided

- 1 (16-ounce) package extra-firm tofu, drained, pressed, and cubed

- 1 cup yellow onion, chopped

- 1 tablespoon fresh ginger, minced

- 2 garlic cloves, minced

- 2 large tomatoes, chopped finely

- 5 cups frozen peas, thawed

- 1 teaspoon white sesame seeds

Directions:

For sauce: in a bowl, add the chili-garlic sauce and soy sauce and mix until well combined.

In a large skillet, heat 1 tablespoon of oil over medium-high heat and cook the tofu for about 4–5 minutes or until browned completely, stirring occasionally.

Transfer the tofu into a bowl.

In the same skillet, heat the remaining oil over medium heat and sauté the onion for about 3–4 minutes.

Add the ginger and garlic and sauté for about 1 minute.

Add the tomatoes and cook for about 4–5 minutes, crushing with the back of spoon.

Stir in all three peas and cook for about 2–3 minutes.

Stir in the sauce mixture and tofu and cook for about 1–2 minutes.

Serve hot with the garnishing of sesame seeds.

Nutrition Info:

Calories 291 Total Fat 11.9 g

Saturated Fat 1.1 g Cholesterol 0 mg

Sodium 732 mg Total Carbs 31.6 g

Fiber 10.8 g Sugar 11.5 g Protein 19 g

Mango Tofu Curry

Servings: 2

Cooking Time: 35 Minutes

Ingredients:

- 1lb cubed extra firm tofu

- 1lb chopped vegetables

- 1 cup low carb mango sauce

- 1 cup vegetable broth

- 2tbsp curry paste

Directions:

Mix all the ingredients in your Instant Pot.

Cook on Stew for 35 minutes.

Release the pressure naturally.

Nutrition Info:

Calories: 310

Carbs: 20

Sugar: 9 Fat: 4

Protein: 37 GL: 19

Dried Fruit Squash

Servings: 4

Cooking Time: 40 Minutes

Ingredients:

- ¼ cup water

- 1 medium butternut squash, halved and seeded

- ½ tablespoon olive oil

- ½ tablespoon balsamic vinegar

- Salt and ground black pepper, to taste

- 4 large dates, pitted and chopped

- 4 fresh figs, chopped

- 3 tablespoons pistachios, chopped

- 2 tablespoons pumpkin seeds

Directions:

Preheat the oven to 375°F.

Place the water in the bottom of a baking dish.

Arrange the squash halves in a large baking dish, hollow-side up, and drizzle with oil and vinegar.

Sprinkle with salt and black pepper.

Spread the dates, figs, and pistachios on top.

Bake for about 40 minutes, or until squash becomes tender.

Serve hot with the garnishing of pumpkin seeds.

Nutrition Info:

Calories 227 Total Fat 5.5 g

Saturated Fat 0.8 g

Cholesterol 0 mg Sodium 66 mg

Total Carbs 46.4 g Fiber 7.5 g

Sugar 19.6 g Protein 5 g

Spiced Couscous Tomatoes

Servings: 8

Cooking Time: 15 Minutes

Ingredients:

- ½ teaspoon cumin, ground

- 1 teaspoon coriander, ground

- 8 beefsteak tomatoes

- ½ cup sliced almonds

- 1 eggplant, cut into ½ inch slices

- What you will need from the store cupboard:

- 1 cup vegetable broth, low-sodium

- 1 tablespoon olive oil

- ½ cup couscous

- 1 teaspoon harissa paste

- Salt and pepper to taste

- Pinch of ground cinnamon

Directions:

Sprinkle some salt inside the hollowed-out tomatoes.

Keep them on a plate, upside down. Use paper towels to cover.

Heat ½ of the olive oil in your saucepan.

Add almonds. Cook for 2-3 minutes over low temperature.

Add the other ingredients to the saucepan.

Stir the eggplant in. Cook while turning until it is tender and brown.

Stir in the cumin, cinnamon, and coriander.

Pour the broth in and boil. Now add the couscous.

Take out from the heat. Keep aside for 5 minutes.

Return to low temperature. Cook for 2 minutes.

Use a fork, separating the couscous grains.

Stir the almonds in and add the harissa paste to the mix.

Pour over the couscous. Season with pepper. Mix well.

Spoon the mixture into your tomatoes.

Nutrition Info:

Calories 175, Fat 6g, Protein 5g, Carbohydrates 28g, Fiber 5g, Cholesterol 0mg, Sugar 1.1g

CPSIA information can be obtained
at www.ICGtesting.com
Printed in the USA
BVHW091517100621
609271BV00004B/930

9 781802 571790